Friend Grief and ANGER:

WHEN YOUR FRIEND DIES AND NO ONE GIVES A DAMN

Victoria Noe

Photograph of Delle Chatman reproduced with permission from Gregory Chatman

Excerpt from *Outrageous Conduct: Art, Ego and The Twilight Zone Case* used with permission by Stephen Farber.

For a list of grief support resources: www.FriendGrief.com

Printed in the United States of America
First Printing, 2013

ISBN 978-0-9884632-1-9
ISBN 978-0-9884632-0-2 (print)

King Company – Chicago, IL 60618

www.FriendGrief.com

Dedication

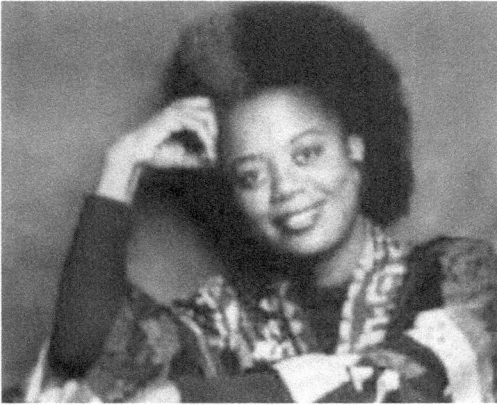

Delle Chatman

To Delle Chatman, who was right as always

Table of Contents

Introduction: The Shock of Anger........................ 1

Who Are You Angry With? 5

Permission to Be Angry 9

"I'm Angry. And I Don't Know What to Do
with My Anger.".. 11

Picking a Scab 17

Angry in Public... 21

AIDS@30: Forming Community........................ 23

Funeral for a Friend..................................... 29

"How Long Has This Been Going On?" 33

It Can Go Either Way................................... 37

What Have We Learned? 41

Acknowledgements...................................... 43

References.. 45

Introduction:
The Shock of Anger

In the spring of 2011, two months after I started my blog, *Friend Grief,* Tracy Baim, publisher of Chicago's oldest gay/lesbian newspaper, *Windy City Times,* asked if I'd contribute to their excellent, year-long series, *AIDS@30.* The series would chronicle the AIDS epidemic from local, national and international perspectives. I'd known her since I worked as a staff and consulting fundraiser in the Chicago AIDS community in the late 80s and early 90s.

The first decade of the epidemic was a frightening time. Ignorance and hate were on constant display. I'd run into people, mostly men, I hadn't seen for a while and cringe when they had "the look." There was a certain look about those with AIDS: emaciated body, dark lesions, haunted eyes.

The weekly gay papers were full of obituaries. The mainstream papers simply attributed the cause of death to 'a long illness' but we knew the truth. For years, our social lives revolved around memorial services and fundraising events. My work was gratifying, but emotionally exhausting.

When I sat down at my computer, I hoped I could remember enough specifics about that time in my life to fill Tracy's guidelines. To my surprise, instead of having trouble remembering, words flew off my fingertips, burning up the keyboard with long-suppressed rage.

"I can name names," I thought to myself. "What difference does it make? They're dead."

I was shocked at the depth of those feelings. I hadn't thought about that time for years, and assumed I'd gotten over the anger long ago. When I first started writing the piece, I wallowed in it, enjoying my self-righteous anger. Gradually I calmed down. But my reaction still surprised me.

Grieving a friend is difficult enough. To compound it, you may also feel that your grief is not respected: that it is, in the words of Dr. Kenneth Doka at the College of New Rochelle, *disenfranchised grief.*

Doka coined the phrase to describe "grief that is not openly acknowledged, socially validated or publicly observed."

Maybe you tried to share your sad news, only to be confronted by people who dismiss it entirely or find it lacking in comparison to their own. They might tell you their grief is more profound than yours – especially if they grieve a family member. Others will tell you they know "just how you feel" because their cat died. I'm not going to debate anyone about the depth of grief they felt when their pet died, much less a relative. But for me, grieving a friend poses its own unique challenges.

Although it happens to us all sooner or later, your grief after the death of your friend may surprise you.

We tend to take our friendships for granted, especially the

long-term ones. Our friends are a part of our lives, and we assume they will just always be there, even if we see them rarely.

We feel all the normal responses to news of a death: shock, disbelief, regret, sadness. The one that may surprise you the most is anger, because it's probably the response that's talked about the least.

In the following pages, we'll look at people whose anger after a friend's death was very real. The focus of the anger varies: sometimes it's directed at what or who killed them, sometimes it's the friend themselves. Sometimes, the deepest anger is reserved for themselves.

These stories will help you acknowledge your anger and be comforted by the fact that you're not alone in this very human response. And they may even help you take the first steps towards moving through that anger.

Like the other stages of grief we hear so much about, anger is normal and natural. And now we're going to admit it.

Who Are You Angry With?

Anger can be unattractive, there's no question about it. It's messy and unpredictable, sometimes loud and violent. And in a world where we like things to make sense, it's often unacceptable. But it's never more unacceptable than when you're grieving. There's a long list of people we can be angry with:

The person who died: Why didn't they take better care of themselves? Why did they take such a stupid chance? What were they thinking?

The medical community: Why didn't the doctor force them to take better care of their health? Why didn't the paramedics get there sooner? Why hasn't someone discovered a cure for cancer, or heart disease?

The family: Why didn't they make him go to the doctor? Why did they let her live alone?

God: Why did you make a good person suffer? Why didn't

you answer their prayers? Why did you leave those children without a parent? Why them? Why now? Why not someone else? Why not me?

Why?

Why?

Why?

Death is, after all, the great unknown. And that mystery makes us scared about what we will face. Despite stories of white lights and visions of deceased relatives, no one's come back from any extended time in the afterlife. We don't know what awaits us.

And we *really* don't know why people die when they do. We say "it was just their time," and obviously, it was. But that doesn't answer *why?* As a friend, that sense of helplessness can create even deeper anger.

Many times when I've grieved I've been angry, although I rarely shared those feelings. I was ashamed of my anger. I felt that admitting it was shifting the focus away from my friend, and onto me. It felt selfish.

Anger can be useful, but when unacknowledged or suppressed it is more likely to present itself as depression. That's not what I'm talking about here. I'm talking about admitting that white-hot, body-shaking, screaming-at-the-top-of-your-lungs rage.

You've already realized that the grief you feel for your friend is being devalued because you're not family. And that can add to the anger you already feel.

Even those who are also grieving are unlikely to understand your anger. Think of Sally Field melting down in the cemetery in *Steel Magnolias*, and the shock on her friends' faces. The minister in *The Big Chill* who says "I'm angry, and I don't know what to do with my anger" is much calmer about it, but the look in his eyes is not.

The problem with suppressing the absolutely justified anger we feel when a friend dies is that it will bubble up eventually. It will present itself suddenly and loudly and often in a completely unrelated situation. And that presents its own complications. Screaming at a barista who doesn't know you may feel momentarily satisfying, but it won't bring back your friend.

So, if you're angry that cancer treatments and cures came too late for your friend...

If you're angry that your friend's family refused to notify you of her death...

If you're angry that your friend drove drunk...

If you're angry that an evil person chose your friend at random to kill...

Accept that anger and embrace it. You're angry because of the pain that your friend's death has caused. That's, dare I say it, normal. Frankly, it would be strange if you weren't angry. You're angry because you loved them and wanted them to stay close to you always. Selfish maybe, but normal and human.

So, as long as you don't hurt yourself or anyone else, you have my permission to be angry. As time goes on, you can work on channeling your anger into positive action, to keep your friend's memory alive every day of your life.

Permission to Be Angry

Unless they take the time to post comments, sometimes it's hard to tell what my blog readers are thinking. But anger has been one of those topics that really resonated with people.

The comment that stuck with me most was the woman who emailed me privately to thank me for giving her permission to be angry.

Imagine: a grown woman who needed a stranger's permission to feel angry. *Why **wouldn't** you feel angry if your friend is dead?*

Yes, of course you're sad. You feel a hole in your heart and your life. But it's ridiculously hard for people – men and women both – to admit anger. Usually, you'll find anger reserved for the person or situation you blame: the doctors, the drunk driver, the cancer. Occasionally, you'll be angry at the friend themselves. Sometimes, you might even be mad at yourself, for not being able to prevent it or for not keeping in touch with your friend.

All of those reasons are valid, if not necessarily accurate. Chances are, there was nothing you could do to change the outcome. Even doctors aren't infallible.

But that anger deserves to be acknowledged and accepted. It deserves to be felt, and needs to be felt, no matter how messy it is.

I'm a firm believer in anger. I think it's easy to get stuck in grief if you've never been angry, or if you dismiss the possibility of anger. It's easy to get mired in grief if you can't get past being angry.

You may be familiar with Elisabeth Kubler-Ross' famous stages of grief: denial, anger, bargaining, depression and acceptance. They were first identified to describe the journey of someone who is dying – but they were later attributed to those who mourn. She did not mean for this to be a complete or chronological list. But anger, like the others, is a *stage*. It's not healthy to suppress anger. And it's not the end of the journey because it's not meant to be a permanent condition.

I'm skeptical of people who insist they've never been angry about the death of a loved one; more likely they haven't gotten there yet. Or maybe they feel ashamed of their anger, thinking it's an inappropriate response.

Well, time's up. Let's meet some angry people.

"I'm Angry. And I Don't Know What to Do with My Anger."

The minister leading the funeral service at the beginning of *The Big Chill* was talking about Alex, the friend whose suicide sets the stage for this hit movie. His sudden death brings a group of friends together for the first time since college. Their initial shock, over the course of their "reunion" weekend, fades to more mundane issues: sex, drugs, purpose in life. But eventually the subject of Alex's suicide bubbles up again, and their grief is expressed in anger: at their friend for not reaching out to them, and themselves for not being able to stop him from ending his life.

"I knew he was unhappy," says one character. Some felt they would've had the power to cheer him up, keep him happy enough to stay alive. Eventually, as they move past their anger and guilt, they have to accept that Alex's decision was not about them. By the end of the movie, some of them decide to use him as a reason/excuse to recommit to their own passions.

Like the characters in *The Big Chill,* we often try to shove aside anger when we grieve, but it persists – and it can push us forward if we deal with it.

One of the consequences of this life is that we experience the deaths of our family and friends. Some of those times are easier to get through. Others are more problematic. My friend, Delle Chatman's death was one of those challenging times that pushed me forward in ways I could never have predicted.

She'd fought recurring ovarian cancer for almost four years, but was in remission Labor Day, 2006. Recent complications, most troubling a sudden build-up of fluid in her lungs, necessitated her hospitalization the weekend before our daughters went back to school.

I had the fortune or misfortune to walk into her room as her doctor walked out. As soon as I did, I knew something was very wrong. The cancer was back again, Delle told me, but this time her reaction and mine were different from previous bouts. This time, there was no immediate assurance from her that this was a mere bump in the road, nor from me, that it would be quickly dispatched. We never said it, exactly, but we both seemed to know.

I sat on her bed while she made phone calls and we made lists – one of my more sought-after skills – of others to call and errands to organize. There were few tears, and as I recall, they were all hers. I was determined not to cry in front of her, mostly because I knew she'd wind up comforting me. Somehow that was unacceptable. Though she always remained fiercely independent, her friends all felt protective of her. We saw our role as keeping her spirits up, not the other way around. I left a couple hours later, just before her daughter was due to arrive.

Northwestern Memorial Hospital is just off Chicago's Magnificent Mile™. A block away from where I left Delle, you are in the midst of shopping, hotels, restaurants, traffic, tourists from around the world. I walked out and headed in that direction, but got only around the corner before I had to stop. I called my husband and said, "The cancer's back. This is different. This is it."

I started walking again, and as I reached Michigan Avenue on that bright, beautiful holiday weekend, I wanted to kill every person I saw on the street. I hated them: every single one. What right did they have to live, to be happy, when my friend was dying?

I was distraught, but mostly I was angry: angry with God, angry with the cancer for returning, angry that the doctors couldn't make it go away permanently, angry with myself for being powerless.

The next month brought a flurry of activity, as Delle went back into treatment. She kept her friends informed of her progress through her Yahoo groups. Her first remission was a miracle, as was the next. Everyone assumed yet another one; everyone but me. I prayed I was wrong, but I still couldn't shake the feeling that this was different.

Delle had gone on retreat twice that summer. Her spirituality was daunting to me: it fueled her in ways that were both inspiring and intimidating. Even when her church gave up on her, she didn't give up on it. She'd been an Augustus Tolton scholar at Catholic Theological, and felt a deep calling to be a priest. Earlier in her illness, the Cardinal, unhappy with her public admission of that calling, told her she had to remain silent, or lose her scholarship and health care. I remember sitting in our favorite coffee house, as she cried over the decision she had to make. In the end, there was no decision: she would not be silenced, and she paid the price.

It was not a surprise. An op-ed piece she wrote for the *Chicago Tribune* emphasized that although the hierarchy of the Church had abandoned her in her desire to become a priest, she remained a Catholic "bone deep". Her spirituality trumped dogma, and I admired her for that.

Now I see that those retreats were her preparation for the dramatic turn of events in the fall. I don't know if she suspected that the end was near or just wanted the strength for whatever happened.

After a month, she announced on her Yahoo groups that she was discontinuing treatment: her body simply couldn't take any more. On election night, 2006, in the company of her friend and caregiver, daughter and brothers, she left us. She was two weeks shy of her 55th birthday.

A few months before she died, I told her my idea for a book about people grieving their friends and she enthusiastically supported it. I'd never written a book before, but her "just do it" was more than a pithy Nike tagline: it was heartfelt.

I knew she meant it. I knew she believed I could do it. But I didn't. I'd had other ideas for books that never saw me put pen to paper. I didn't believe in myself, even though she did. It would take a while for me to be convinced.

On Christmas Day, 2009, I was in St. Louis at mass with my best friend and my family. I'd had a rough year, enduring physical and emotional challenges that brought me to my knees more than once. And although the book was finally beginning to take shape, I was in the midst of a crisis of faith: in myself, those around me, and God. I hoped going to a different church – Sts. Clare & Francis Ecumenical Catholic Communion – would help.

I sat there watching a woman priest concelebrate the mass and saw the same look of joy I'd seen on Delle's face when she spoke of her own never-realized calling. I couldn't hold back the tears, and my head dropped. "That should be you up there on the altar," I imagined myself saying to Delle, sad and angry at the same time. Then I felt arms around me, as if from someone kneeling behind me, though no one was there. Within that embrace, I heard Delle's voice whisper, "it's okay."

It was not the first time I'd felt Delle's presence since she died, nor would it be the last. The tears dried up and I felt a peace I hadn't felt in close to a year, maybe even longer.

My anger over Delle's death has subsided for the most part, although I'm still unable to forgive those who were cruel to her, like the other moms at school who deliberately and illegally parked in the handicapped space that she needed. What I'm left with, finally, is gratitude. I can't imagine what my life would be like now, having made a huge career change to writing, without her encouragement and inspiration.

On those days when I'm most frustrated and distracted, obsessing about money or some perceived injustice, if I'm really quiet I can hear Delle's voice: "if you'd write the damn book, you wouldn't have to worry about that."

I am writing it, and I hope she likes it. If not, I'm pretty sure I'll hear about it.

Picking a Scab

My blog posts about feeling angry dredged up feelings for many readers that had been long suppressed. The validation of their anger gave them the freedom to respond with great emotion.

Some people took the opportunity to fondly remember a friend. Others reacted as if a scab had been scratched, and indeed it had. Those were the people who had been denied the chance to feel that anger when their friend died, and now, years later, it bubbled up again.

You can only hold your breath so long, and eventually you have to breathe again. So it is with emotions. Eventually they decide they've been constrained long enough.

Those who are overwhelmed by sudden, intense feelings of anger share another feeling: powerlessness. They are unable to reconcile what happened to their friend, to what they believe is the natural order of the universe. How else can you explain comments such as:

"They shouldn't have died."

"It doesn't make any sense."

"I just talked to her."

"They weren't even supposed to be there."

They want to believe things are supposed to happen a certain way; in fact, they're desperate to believe it.

If there is an order to the universe, then their friend shouldn't have died.

They can only accept that their friend died if there's a reasonable, logical explanation. If they had to die, there has to be a reason. And it has to be an extraordinarily good reason.

Perhaps their diagnosis alerted people to the consequences of using tanning beds, or ignoring warning signs of heart disease. Perhaps their friend died in the line of duty saving someone else. First responders deal with the possibility of death every day, but their friends may forget that fact.

As we all know, often there is no explanation, reasonable or otherwise.

That's where anger pops up.

I don't know if God is flippant enough to insist, "Because I said so," when asked why someone had to die. And I don't know if there's a more irritating phrase than "it was just their time."

I've had friends who died from enemy gunfire and cancer, car accidents and suicide, AIDS and the 9/11 attacks. Not one of those deaths made sense to me. Not one of those friends deserved to suffer – sometimes for years, sometimes for seconds. Not one of those deaths could be justified in my mind as being necessary.

But all forced me to admit that I could not change what had happened, and for a control freak, that's a tough lesson.

We're all control freaks when it comes to death. We have no control over the circumstances of our birth and very little over the circumstances of our death. And since we tend to be adults when the second one happens, we believe we should have a say: not only about our own deaths, but about those of the people we love.

If possible, all of us would do whatever was in our power to spare our friend's suffering and death. Love does that: it makes you want to protect the ones you love. The hardest lesson of all is that, ultimately, you can't.

But instead of throwing a much-deserved tantrum because we have no power, we have to sit back and say, "I hate that this happened to my friend. I hate it with every breath I take. But I can't change it, and that kills me, a little, too."

That tantrum probably feels very satisfying – at least in my experience it does. But it has to be followed by Kubler-Ross's stage of acceptance. Acceptance doesn't imply enthusiasm or even closure. In fact, acceptance may feel more like surrender.

That's when we have to decide how we want to remember that friend: by how they died, or how they lived? What part of them will we hold in our hearts for the rest of our lives? What part of them will inspire us and motivate us?

Take, for example, John F. Kennedy and Martin Luther King, Jr. Both were assassinated, and that's the day we chose to remember Kennedy. But in the case of Dr. King, it's his birthday, January 15. It's become a national holiday and day of service.

I don't know why JFK's memory hasn't inspired this type of response, but it points out two very different ways of remembering someone.

So, have your rant. Scream, yell, cry; try not to hurt yourself or anyone nearby. Have it out, once and for all. You need that physical release to respond to the stress of your friend's death.

Then decide how your friend will guide you. That's something you do have power over.

Angry in Public

Let's take that anger a step further, to a situation most of us will not face after the death of a friend.

Perhaps your friend, though not a public figure, died in a way that attracts media attention: they died of AIDS, on 9/11, in Afghanistan or a horrific car accident.

Perhaps your friend was a public figure: a politician, professional athlete, musician or actor. They were used to intense public scrutiny.

Either way, now they're dead, and they have no control over what is said and written about their life and death. While their family may have legal recourse, as their friend, you have none. You must listen to the commentators and pseudo-friends describe your friend in ways that anger you. Maybe your friend was doing something risky when they died, like race car driver Dale Whedon, who was killed in a horrific crash in 2011. But that doesn't mean they did it because they wanted to die.

This dissecting of lives in the public eye will not go away any time soon. Celebrity deaths are big business: not just tabloids and TV specials, but commemorative magazines, limited edition collector plates and cemetery tours.

The 911 calls placed when a celebrity is found dead – Michael Jackson comes to mind – are played and replayed on TV. Autopsy photos are leaked. Onlookers who witnessed the suicide of film director Tony Scott taped his leap off a Los Angeles bridge. Then they shopped it around to websites and media outlets.

Interesting? Something you'd want to watch or listen to or read about? Now imagine if they were a friend of yours: still as interesting?

We also assume that celebrities are always "on": ready to make a statement to the media on any topic. But when asked to respond to the news of John Lennon's murder, former Beatle Paul McCartney did not have an eloquent response. The world criticized him for saying only, "It's a drag." It certainly looks like a less-than-adequate response in print. The video of his comment, though, shows a man at a loss for words to describe his grief.

For years afterwards, McCartney was asked to justify or explain his reaction. But he can't. By his own admission, he still can't put his feelings into words: this from a man who's penned the lyrics to some of the most memorable songs in rock and roll history.

The next time you're tempted to gossip about a recently-deceased celebrity, remember: they left behind family and friends who are doing their grieving in public.

AIDS@30:
Forming Community

The first time I remember being conscious of the effects of AIDS was March, 1983. My girlfriend was in the hospital, after a difficult labor and delivery that called for a transfusion. She worked in the lab at that hospital and knew the blood supply wasn't safe. When I visited her there, her skin was whiter than her sheets. But she refused the transfusion until her doctor finally convinced her.

During the 80's, I volunteered in the AIDS community occasionally, mostly to help raise money. In 1989, I took a job as development director at Chicago House, a residential and support service for men and women living with AIDS. I was the only straight person in the office, a fact that did not meet with universal approval.

The animosity directed towards me as a straight woman in the AIDS community surprised me. AIDS was still considered a gay issue, and there was a bit of territorialism. The gay community was mostly on its own: they not only had to fight for every dollar, but they had to fight prejudice at the same time. I suppose I was naïve. I had no agenda; I just wanted to help.

I came from a theatre background, so I'd had gay friends since high school (even wound up dating a couple, unintentionally). However, so many of the guys I went to school with have died, many of them from AIDS, that I've never been to a college reunion. I didn't want to hear about any more. I found out one of them died when I saw his panel on the cover of a book about the Names Project AIDS Memorial Quilt.

There was a constant stream of fundraisers in those days: bar events at Little Jim's and Roscoe's, drag shows, a dunk tank at Halsted Street Days, and our first black-tie event at the Drake Hotel. I was in London the year before I started at Chicago House on the first World AIDS Day, and a collection was taken up at curtain call in the West End theatres. I stole that idea the following year, and we sent volunteers to theatres to collect money for Chicago House. Some of those volunteers have remained treasured friends to this day.

I left Chicago House after a year and continued to raise money in the AIDS community as a consultant with groups like Bonaventure House and Stop AIDS. But there was a price to pay, and it was an emotional one.

I went through as stretch of eleven weeks in a row, where someone I knew died every week. Only one was really close, Steve Showalter, who'd been my assistant at Chicago House. But all were men I'd known around the community, had worked with on projects, or just knew socially.

When I heard about the eleventh one, I called my former acting teacher in L.A. and asked if I could visit. I booked a seat on Amtrak: two days with no phones, and no contact with others unless I wanted it.

In times of great stress, I need to retreat into myself. I needed the solitude of that long train ride, cutting myself off from the world. I listened to tapes on my Walkman – Beatles, Phil Collins, Crosby, Stills, Nash & Young – music that would soothe and eventually revive me. I read murder mysteries and magazines I didn't normally read, immersing myself in mindless articles about celebrities and fashion that made no mention of AIDS. By the time I got to Los Angeles, I was able to hold a coherent conversation; by the time I came back a week later, I could work again.

As soon as it came out, I bought a copy of *And the Band Played On*, Randy Shilts' indictment of pretty much everyone in the 80s. There are a few heroes in his book, but no end of villains: unethical researchers, an indifferent government, media hysteria. I remember very clearly throwing the book across my living room several times. I'd read about government inaction, or medical fraud, or politics, and I'd have to stop – to throw the book. I've considered buying a copy that wasn't so beat up, but I think I want to hold on to that reminder of my anger. Someone asked recently why I read it when I'd already lived through it. The anger: that's why. Part of me feels that if I'm not angry, I'll forget the people who died.

But often I didn't need to call forth the anger. Now and then, I'd mention going to a memorial service, visiting someone at one of the AIDS wards, or referring someone to Herdegen-Brieske Funeral Home (one of the few in Chicago that would handle arrangements for those who died of AIDS), and I would be asked "How did they get it?" There were few things – then or since – that could instantly infuriate me like that question. My responses were not exactly polite. The nicest I could come up with was "What the hell difference does it make?"

Looking back on that time, I was angry a lot. I felt as if I was living in London during the Blitz: never knowing where the bombs would drop, only knowing that someone I knew would die. A lot of people felt those deaths were deserved: God's punishment for an immoral lifestyle. They were less judgmental if the victim was an "innocent" child or a woman. But even worse, in my eyes, was that most people just didn't care that my friends were dying, because they considered my friends to be somehow inferior.

There are those who feel an ownership to the AIDS crisis, and I understand that. There was certainly a lot of suspicion and occasional antagonism towards any "breeders" (straight people) who joined the efforts. The gay community was devastated, and my losses, though important to me, paled in comparison.

I never imagined that thirty years later there would still be no vaccine, no cure, and there would be new infections every day, even in the gay community. I wonder if what I did made any difference, as if I could've single-handedly cured AIDS. I've had to come to peace with the idea that while I didn't discover a vaccine, I did what I was able to do.

In those years, I grew accustomed to worry and old habits die hard – thirty years later I worry about my gay nephew, even though he assures me he practices safe sex. I worry about my gay friends who have been HIV-positive for decades, healthy thanks to the efficacy of the AIDS cocktail of drugs. I worry about my gay friends who I know are HIV-negative, because I'm just used to worrying about them. And I'm occasionally angry that AIDS is still a cause for worry.

I remember a moment in the early 80's when I thought to

myself: "I don't want to look back and be ashamed I stood by and did nothing."

What I did wasn't much, and it may not have changed anything. My friends are still dead, and I'll probably lose more to this horrible disease. But I'd do it again, gladly, even knowing I'd lose so many people I cared about.

Funeral for a Friend

It's certainly an unusual situation: to be at a funeral with the person you hold responsible for your friend's death.

A friend of mine is among a group of men who worked together on a popular 60s TV show, *Combat!*: Vic Morrow, Rick Jason, Jack Hogan, Pierre Jalbert, Dick Peabody. Talented men who loved playing "soldier" and remained friends after the series was cancelled in 1967.

Vic Morrow's career had its ups and downs, but he was the most well-known of the group. And when he was killed along with two child actors on the set of *Twilight Zone: The Movie* in 1982, all the news stories mentioned *Combat!*.

Controversy about the circumstances of Morrow's death erupted immediately, with many people believing negligence on the part of director John Landis (he was later acquitted of manslaughter in a well-publicized trial). There was no confusion in the minds of Morrow's friends: they blamed Landis.

They were livid about how Morrow's participation in the film was portrayed: that he was excited about it and saw it as a new start for his career.

In fact, Morrow was concerned about safety issues, but didn't feel he could risk quitting the film.

Dick Peabody recalled the anger felt at the funeral in this reflection in the *Mountain Democrat* (Placerville, California), in 1991:

> Moments after we arrived, an audible shock wave of reaction from Vic's friends and co-workers who came to pay their respects, grabbed my attention.
>
> A thin, bearded man was coming down the aisle, seemingly unable to walk without assistance. He was supported by a woman and another man (Mrs. John Landis and George Folsey, Jr., the production manager of the *Twilight Zone* movie). The bearded staggerer was *Twilight Zone* director, John Landis.
>
> His stooges helped him to the lectern and he began a rambling eulogy – unplanned, unrequested, unwanted and shocking to Vic's family and friends. His mere presence at the funeral was offensive to them.

George Folsey, Jr. was asked by his friend, Barbara Turner (Morrow's ex-wife and mother of their daughters, Carrie Morrow and Jennifer Jason-Leigh) to give one of the eulogies. He'd known Turner for years, but had only met Morrow when filming began on *Twilight Zone*. They'd become fast friends. Morrow's former cast mates weren't the only ones outraged at the funeral, as recounted in *Outrageous Conduct: Art, Ego and the Twilight Zone Case*:

When Vic's close friend Steve Shagan arrived at the chapel, he was distressed to learn that both Folsey and Landis planned to deliver eulogies. Still in a state of shock himself, Shagan felt that the funeral service should have the dignity that Vic's horrific death had lacked. When Shagan indicated his objections, Folsey asked Shagan to listen to the remarks he had prepared.

Shagan was appalled by the self-serving testimonial. "Why don't you just run the trailer?" he screamed at Folsey. "Let's set up a screen right here. We can even sell tickets."

Folsey tried to defend the appropriateness of the speech he had written.

"You're not going to read that thing," Shagan countered irately. "If you want to say he worked hard, that's up you and his daughters. But don't talk about that fucking movie! Jesus Christ, there has to be a time and place where somebody isn't selling tickets."

Eventually Folsey was prevailed upon to abbreviate his talk. Would Morrow's friends and family have felt better if John Landis and George Folsey, Jr. had not come to the funeral? Would a conviction for Landis and Folsey have provided closure? I don't know. I don't believe in closure. But I hope to never come face to face with anyone responsible for a friend's death. Like one of Morrow's former cast mates, I'm pretty sure I'd have to be restrained.

"How Long Has This Been Going On?"

Carol Storm was a popular Chicago actress. She was probably best known for portraying Mayor Jane Byrne in *Byrne Baby Byrne III: Whatever Happened to Baby Jane?* We got to know each when we served on the board of directors of a small theatre company. Board meetings were never dull. With Carol there, you cut to the chase: no long-winded speeches, no half-baked defenses of your position.

She was a brusque, sometimes intimidating personality, who did not suffer fools gladly. She demanded honesty and action, but only because she delivered both herself. A compliment from Carol was high praise. You wanted her to be your friend because you certainly didn't want her opposing you for any reason.

Although she wasn't what one would call a party animal, after her breast cancer diagnosis she became even more private. Her friends wanted to help, but she didn't want our help, She preferred to rely only on her partner.

As her condition worsened, she set very strict parameters: no one could visit her, and she would only talk to three people on the phone. For reasons I still don't understand – because we weren't all that close – I was one of the three.

We spoke very little about her health. She would give minimal answers to questions, rarely going into detail, except to prove her determination to flout the no-smoking rules at Northwestern Memorial Hospital. We talked of many things, any things. I remember in particular a call from her one night. She'd been watching Congressional hearings on C-SPAN.

"How long has this been going on?" she demanded.

"I don't know," I replied, "a few weeks?"

"No, not that: how long has C-SPAN been going on?"

It was as if she'd discovered the pot of gold at the end of the rainbow. I have no doubt she saw it as theatre. She loved the gavel to gavel, no-commentary coverage; she was more than capable of providing her own.

I was visiting my parents for Christmas, 1991, when I got a call from my friend, Beth, telling me that Carol had died.

Maybe because we couldn't see her, could only hear her voice on the phone, we'd convinced ourselves that she'd eventually be fine. We knew she didn't want to die, and the recounting by her partner of Carol's last hours proved that she fought right up to the end.

Some funerals are bad because of the circumstances of the death; others are bad because of the age of the person who died. Carol's wake was the first time I ever felt real anger in a funeral home. It was not my first funeral. She was not my first friend to die. But she was the first dead friend I was angry with.

A group of us sat in the back of the parlor, and you would be hard pressed to find a more angry collection of friends. We were angry she was dead, angry the cancer killed her. But we were also angry at Carol.

She'd shut us out, and that was her right. We knew we couldn't cure her cancer or save her life. But we were egotistical enough to believe that we could have made some difference in her struggle, if only she'd let us. We would've all jumped at the chance to visit with her, drive her to the doctor, hold her hand.

But she wouldn't let us.

We lost the chance to help in any little way we could. And we'd lost the chance to say goodbye.

It Can Go Either Way

Washington, DC was in the midst of a sweltering heat wave in early July, 2012. But the Smithsonian Folkways Festival on the National Mall was not cancelled. The triple-digit heat index each day may have affected the numbers of people who came out, but not their passion.

Part of the Festival commemorated the 25th anniversary of the AIDS Memorial Quilt. "Creativity and Crisis" programs and performances addressed the arts community's response to the AIDS epidemic.

The Names Project/AIDS Memorial Quilt – now over 48,000 panels with more than 94,000 names – is still a growing, living memorial to the men, women and children who died from this still incurable disease. But no one – no one – who attended that first organizing meeting in June, 1987, in the Castro district of San Francisco, believed it would still be displayed and growing twenty-five years later.

No one thought long-term, because in the 1980s, there was no long-term for those who contracted the AIDS virus. Life expectancy was measured in weeks and months.

The AIDS Quilt is a very public, very dramatic example of how we can channel our anger into action after the death of a friend. The impulse for its creation was simple: to put a face on the epidemic, to remember those who died, to make sure they were not forgotten. Creating the panels helped the quilters work through their grief, and keep a connection to those who had died.

The Quilt, though, as a response to the epidemic, probably lies at one end of the spectrum. Though initially confrontational (one panelist spoke of the first display on the National Mall as "laying their bodies in front of the government"), it was a way to face their grief and anger, as another panelist insisted, "with love."

At the other end of the spectrum was the AIDS Coalition to Unleash Power (ACT UP): militant, in-your-face, loud, relentless. They channeled their anger into – anger. Certainly, people who were less confrontational gravitated towards the quilt. But by the fall of 1988, 1,000 people had died of AIDS just in San Francisco. What we knew about transmission and treatment was minimal. Fear was palpable. People were dying every day, and no one knew how to slow it down, much less stop it. The worst part for those who were dying, and those who loved them, was that most people outside their community just didn't care.

What ACT UP did – incredibly successfully – was force the issue. Remember: time was not on their side. They were fueled by necessity as well as anger directed at our government, the medical community and the world at large. Vito Russo, activist and author of *The Celluloid Closet*, who later died of AIDS, eloquently described what it was like to be him in his testimony at the Department of Health and Human Services on October 10, 1988:

> Living with AIDS is like living through a war which is happening only for those people who happen to be in the trenches. Every time a shell explodes, you look around and you discover that you've lost more of your friends, but nobody else notices. It isn't happening to them. They're walking the streets as though we weren't living through some sort of nightmare. And only you can hear the screams of the people who are dying and their cries for help. No one else seems to be noticing.

Every movement – civil rights, peace, equal rights, women's rights – has extremists and moderates. Where you fall on the spectrum depends on how close you are to the issue, and what you consider the most effective response.

So, what can we make of these two wildly different responses? Are they at odds? Can you do both? Actually, you can. A panelist spoke with great affection of a young woman who was an early volunteer. She would literally change out of her black ACT UP shirt and into her white Names Project shirt when she came to their office to work on the Quilt.

One group was focused on change: change in government policies and funding, change in society, change in medical treatment, desperately needed to save lives.

One group was focused on bringing people together to honor and remember their loved ones.

Both were valid ways to channel their grief.

Both were necessary at that time – and now – to focus on

those who were suffering and those who had died.
    And both continue to be successful.

What Have We Learned?

I hope the stories you just read will remind you that...

- **You're not alone. The grief you felt when your friend died – and the anger that goes with it – is something we'll all face one day, and many times over.**

- **You're not devaluing your family. You don't have to share DNA or be related by marriage to love someone. Grief, as they say, is the price you pay for love. Whether we say it out loud or not, we do love our friends.**

- **You're not weird. You can grieve a friend you weren't all that close to, even one you haven't seen in years. You can grieve a celebrity you've never met. It may not make sense to others, but that doesn't mean your grief isn't real.**

- **Last, but certainly not least, your anger is normal, a natural part of the grieving process.**

What matters now – to you and the legacy of your friend-ship – is what you do with that anger.

Accept it.

Face it.

Embrace it.

Then move on, in ways that would make your friend proud.

Acknowledgements

To those whose stories appear in this book: for being honest and sharing their stories.

To my readers: David Beckwith, Kathy Pooler, Ann Smith, Karl Sprague and Kristie West for their honest and constructive suggestions.

To my writing group: Jo Stewart, Penny Savage, Helene Johannessen and Alice Faeth, for their ongoing support, encouragement and inspiration.

To my industry mentors: There are many, but Porter Anderson, Dan Blank, Nina Amir, Eileen Dreyer and Jane Friedman in particular, for guiding me through the maze.

To my editor: Melissa Wuske, and designer, Rebecca Swift, who made it painless and rewarding.

To John and Emma: for your patience.

To all of them, my thanks.

References

Doka, K.J., ed. *Disenfranchised Grief:*
New Directions, Challenges, and Strategies for Practice.
Champaign, IL: Research Press, 2002.

Farber, Stephen, and Marc Green, *Outrageous Conduct:*
Art, Ego and the Twilight Zone Case.
New York: Arbor House, 1988.

LaBrecque, Ron. *Special Effects:*
Disaster at "Twilight Zone": The Tragedy and the Trial.
New York: Charles Scribner's Sons, 1988.

Some of the material in this book was previously published on the following websites and publications:

www.FriendGrief.com

www.windycitymediagroup.com

**Coming Soon:
Book #2 in the Friend Grief series –**

*Friend Grief and AIDS:
Thirty Years of Burying Our Friends*

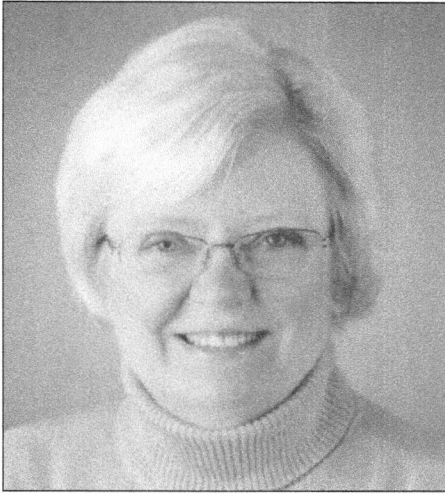

Victoria Noe has been a writer most of her life, but didn't admit it until 2009. After earning a Masters from the University of Iowa in Speech & Dramatic Art, she moved to Chicago, where she worked professionally as a stage manager, director and administrator, as well as a founding board member of the League of Chicago Theatres. Her next career was as a professional fundraiser, raising money for arts, educational and AIDS service organizations. After a concussion ended a successful sales career, she switched gears to keep a promise to a friend to write a book. Her freelance articles have appeared in *Chicago Tribune* and *Windy City Times*. She also reviews books on BroadwayWorld.com. Victoria lives in Chicago with her family.